Intermittent Fasting

7 Effective Techniques with Scientific Approach To Stay Healthy, Lose Weight, Slow Down Aging Process & Live Longer

Stephen Fleming

Copyright © 2017 Stephen Fleming

All rights reserved.

From the Author's Desk

Hi, I am Stephen Fleming and welcome to my book. As one famous CEO stated that life is like juggling three balls of health, family & career and first two balls are made of glass. It can't be restored once broken. So the transformation of life begins with focusing on great health. This book will teach you about 7 practical ways of Intermittent Fasting that could be followed in day to day life to achieve your weight loss & eventually fitness goals. You can choose any one or combination of 7 proposed techniques for your specific requirement. "The idea is to give offer you doable techniques based on my experience & results, which would contribute to your fitness goals and ultimately make you happy! One more thing, if you are suffering from any existing ailments /disease; please consult your physician first. I would really appreciate if you can provide your genuine feedback on amazon after going through the book.

Wishing you lots of health, happiness and success!

Cheers!

Intermittent Fasting: 7 Effective Techniques with scientific approach

Welcome On-Board: Get the FREE BONUS

I am privileged to have you onboard. You have shown faith in me and I would like to reciprocate it by offering the maximum value with an amazing gift.

As you are working towards improving your life consistently, I would like to contribute in your journey by offering a free bonus called "Health & Wealth Magnetism- Using the law of attraction to create Health & Wealth". It provides an interesting perspective to overall success and how health & wealth compliments each other to create a lasting success. I would be adding to this free bonus as I find other beneficial topics that can help contribute in our progress.

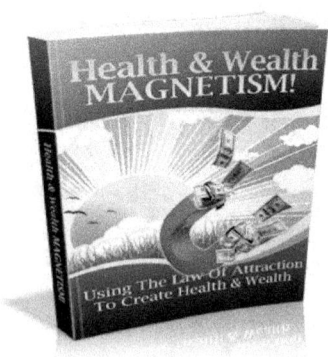

Intermittent Fasting: 7 Effective Techniques with scientific approach

Type this link:
http://eepurl.com/dglqCH

or scan below from your mobile

Intermittent Fasting: 7 Effective Techniques with scientific approach

☐ **Copyright 2017- All rights reserved.**

This document is geared towards providing exact and reliable information in regards to the topic and issue covered. The publication is sold with the idea that the publisher is not required to render accounting, officially permitted, or otherwise, qualified services. If advice is necessary, legal or professional, a practiced individual in the profession should be ordered.

- From a Declaration of Principles which was accepted and approved equally by a Committee of the American Bar Association and a Committee of Publishers and Associations. In no way is it legal to reproduce, duplicate, or transmit any part of this document in either electronic means or in printed format. Recording of this publication is strictly prohibited and any storage of this document is not allowed unless with written permission from the publisher. All rights reserved.

The information provided herein is stated to be truthful and consistent, in that any liability, in terms of inattention or otherwise, by any usage or abuse of any policies, processes, or directions contained within is the solitary and utter responsibility of the recipient reader. Under no circumstances will any legal responsibility or blame be held against the publisher for any reparation, damages, or monetary loss due to the information herein, either directly or indirectly.

Intermittent Fasting: 7 Effective Techniques with scientific approach

Respective authors own all copyrights not held by the publisher. The information herein is offered for informational purposes solely, and is universal as so. The presentation of the information is without contract or any type of guarantee assurance. The trademarks that are used are without any consent, and the publication of the trademark is without permission or backing by the trademark owner. All trademarks and brands within this book are for clarifying purposes only and are the owned by the owners themselves, not affiliated with this document.

Intermittent Fasting: 7 Effective Techniques with scientific approach

CONTENTS

1	Introduction	1
2	Intermittent Fasting Explained	2-4
3	Scientific Logic Behind Intermittent Fasting	5-6
4	Benefits of Intermittent Fasting	7-8
5	Intermittent Fasting Techniques	9-17
6	Tips to Succeed with Fasting & Conclusion	18-20

Intermittent Fasting: 7 Effective Techniques with scientific approach

1. INTRODUCTION

I want to thank you and congratulate you for downloading the book, "Intermittent Fasting - 7 Effective Techniques with Scientific Approach To Stay Healthy, Lose Weight, Slow Down Aging Process & Live Longer"

Did you know that human beings have been fasting since evolution? Basically, human beings mainly fasted due to lack of food and for a number of reasons. For instance, both the ancient man and the hunter-gatherers didn't have food stores or refrigerators to make food available all-year round. In some instances, these people never found anything to eat and their body nevertheless "evolved" to function without food for long periods!

On the other hand, there are religions among them Christians, Islam, and Buddhists who embrace fasting as part of the doctrine. This clearly shows that fasting is not something new. However, how can you exactly fast to lose weight? This is what this book will be about.

This book will teach you about intermittent

Intermittent Fasting: 7 Effective Techniques with scientific approach

fasting, how to lose weight with intermittent fasting, why intermittent fasting is effective at weight loss, 7 techniques of intermittent fasting and so much more.

Thanks again for downloading this book. I hope you enjoy it!

2. INTERMITTENT FASTING EXPLAINED

Intermittent fasting refers to a pattern of eating that alternates between periods of fasting and non-fasting, intended to facilitate weight loss or boost health. For starters, intermittent fasting does not restrict foods or calories to eat but rather suggests when you should eat them.

There are different approaches to intermittent fasting with some involving calorie restriction, skipping some meals and total fasting. For instance, during the fasting period, you can eat limited amounts of low-calories foods or drinks such as tea or coffee. Alternatively, you may choose to reduce intake of calories say to 20 percent on fasting days rather than not eating altogether. If desired, you can also choose to fast for a complete 24 hours then eat normally for the next 24 hours in what is called alternate day fasting.

Due to these flexibilities, it's easier to adopt a favorite dieting plan by deciding the number of hours or days to fast and activities to carry out during the fast. But with too much freedom,

Intermittent Fasting: 7 Effective Techniques with scientific approach

how does intermittent fasting work? Basically, you should understand what happens to your body during the eating phase and the fasted state.

Once you eat, your body is said to be at a fed state where it's digesting and assimilating food and nutrients. The fed state normally commences once you start to eat, and often lasts for 3-5 hours. In this state, it's harder to burn fat due to high levels of insulin.

Insulin is a hormone that facilitates uptake of glucose into body cells. After a high carb meal, glucose level increases which triggers high concentration of insulin. As the hormone only helps glucose uptake, your body has to utilize glucose for energy rather than stored fats.

After the action of insulin, the body goes into post-absorption state where no food is processed, a period that lasts for 8-12 hours after a meal. Then you enter into a fasted state about 12 hours after your last meal, where insulin level is significantly reduced. In a fasted state, it's easier to burn fat that was inaccessible during the period of eating. While there are different intermittent fasting techniques, there are common guidelines applicable across board. Let us look at these guidelines in the following chapter.

Intermittent Fasting Guidelines

According to research, even eating three meals a day can be "eating too much" as far as calorie restriction and meal planning is concerned. The study found out that eating fewer meals a day could be better than increased meal frequency particularly in the long term.

While eating 5-6 smaller meals a day can help control blood sugar and curb hunger, your metabolism often is accustomed to the schedule within 1-2 months. Later on you start experiencing hunger throughout the day rather than around lunch or dinnertime.

A better approach is to embrace intermittent fasting and limit meals to a narrow window of 8 hours ideally by skipping breakfast. To make it easier, choose to either eat breakfast or dinner but not both. For instance you could choose to eat a solid breakfast and lunch if working in a physically taxing job and then skip dinner. The great thing is that it actually

Intermittent Fasting: 7 Effective Techniques with scientific approach

doesn't matter what meal you skip as long as you skip one of the meals.

The rule of the thumb is to only eat within a window of 6-8 consecutive hours daily and then eat meals at least 3 hours before bed. While you can still fast for 24 hours, skipping just a few meals can optimize your mitochondrial function and inhibit any cellular

damage. You don't have to starve yourself but rather eat enough food while allowing the body to rest from constant feeding

In the following chapter, we are going to look at the scientific logic behind intermittent fasting and its effectiveness.

3. SCIENTIFIC LOGIC BEHIND INTERMITTENT FASTING

Whether you simply take coffee for breakfast in place of high-fructose fruit smoothie or skip breakfast altogether, you gain in terms of improved health and weight loss. And while lack of food may be thought to trigger breakdown of muscle, your body first breaks down stored glycogen into glucose to fuel metabolic activities. Once glycogen levels are depleted, the body begins to break down stored fat for energy. In some cases, excess amino acids from proteins can be metabolized for energy though this does not mean the body may break down muscle.

Most people against intermittent fasting state that it reduces your metabolism because your body thinks that you are starving; hence, slowing down, which can make weight loss impossible. However, this is not the case. According to research, the rate of metabolism doesn't change when you enter into a fasting state as long as you don't exceed 60 hours. However, even after 60 hours of continuous fasting, the study found out that the rate of metabolism only reduced by a mere 8 percent.

Intermittent Fasting: 7 Effective Techniques with scientific approach

Actually, to some extent, the rate of metabolism can significantly be speeded up after 36-48 hours of fasting according to related research. This is because when you fast, the brain releases chemicals or neurotransmitters such as adrenaline and noradrenalin. These help activate your mind and basal metabolic rate (BMR) which serves to facilitate you to work or go to search for food. This can continue until 72 hours of total fasting, where the body opts to break down muscle as primary source of energy. In addition to a boosted metabolism, other studies reveal that the intermittent fasting helps boost energy production, memory, and cognitive function. Furthermore, it can boost production of proteins that stimulates neuron growth and protection. This is referred to as neurotrophic growth factor.

Another study found out that intermittent fasting could reduce insulin resistance. An increase in insulin sensitivity and reduced blood pressure help control diseases such as stroke and coronary artery disease. Intermittent fasting can also boost resistance of the heart and brain cells to ischemic injury that causes diseases such as stroke. In a related research, believers who undertake Ramadan fasting were found to have reduced risk to diabetes, improved immunity and cardiovascular health. Though this study was

Intermittent Fasting: 7 Effective Techniques with scientific approach

based on short-term achievements, it's agreed that intermittent fasting is a great thing to try out.

If intending to lose weight or burn fat, a certain study found out that fasting boosts the activity in genes that burn calories and stored body fat. When fasting, the body activates genes that encode enzymes and uncoupling proteins that increase fat oxidation. These proteins "poke holes" into mitochondria (body cells that make energy) and this reduces the overall amount of energy generated. As a result, the body has to burn more fat or calories to achieve the same amount of energy.

Better still; further studies suggest that intermittent fasting can help your cells to handle stress. When you stop eating, body cells are jolted into a minor stressful state, which strengthens them to fight other stresses that often lead to disease.

From the scientific studies, it's obvious that intermittent fasting can help you lose weight, boost cardiovascular health and help you live longer. Let's learn more about these benefits and other benefits of intermittent fasting.

4. BENEFITS OF INTERMITTENT FASTING

Intermittent fasting boasts of benefits such as weight loss, slowing down aging and prolonging your life. Whatever your intended reason for intermittent fasting, you can enjoy a number of benefits like:

1: Weight loss

As already pointed out above, research has shown that people who eat a single meal daily rather than the usual 3 meals lose more weight and have more muscle. This is because dieters who adopt intermittent fasting eat less frequently, actually feel hungry less, and are more likely to feel fuller after eating.

Intermittent fasting can also help you enter a fat burning state referred to as ketosis. When fasting, you deplete your body of glucose, its main source of energy, and this forces the body to break down stored fats for energy. Furthermore, adding MCT oil in coffee during fasting days helps speed up the ketosis process, and yields higher ketones, which fuel the brain.

That's not all; intermittent fasting can be used

as a calorie restriction strategy where you fast for 24 hours at least twice per week. If you follow this eating pattern, you reduce your calorie intake by around 30 percent and thus make it easier to lose weight. By taking in lesser

calories, you force the body to utilize stored glycogen and body fats for energy, a situation that facilitates weight loss.

2: Better hormonal function

Intermittent fasting helps improve your body composition and boosts functionality of hormones. More importantly, you become more sensitive to insulin hormone especially if you pair fasting with exercise. A controlled insulin level helps reduce blood sugar, suppress hunger, and fight occasional food cravings. In addition, research shows that by fasting intermittently for around 40 hours, you also boost the production of growth hormone (GH) up to 5-folds. This hormone has many benefits among them speeding up the rate of fat loss and muscle gain. The growth hormone also helps offset the effects of cortisol, a stress hormone that affects fat storage at the belly.

3: Living longer

Research shows that intermittent fasting can prolong your lifespan in a similar manner as a calorie-restricted diet. This study has found out that reducing your calorie consumption by about 30-40 percent can help extend life at least by 33 percent. Further research shows that fasting can offer health benefits against diabetes, cancer, cardiovascular problems, and Alzheimer's disease among others. A related study found out cancer patients who did alternate day fasting realize better cure rates, which reduced cases of deaths.

Besides all the above benefits, intermittent fasting is also easy to follow given that it makes your day much simpler. For instance, after waking up, you don't have to prepare breakfast but only require a cup of water to kick start the day.

When you're eating one less meal, you're able to plan and prepare less food, which saves time and resources. This simplicity has made intermittent fasting, an effective strategy for

Intermittent Fasting: 7 Effective Techniques with scientific approach

weight loss particularly in obese adults.

With all these benefits you stand to benefit, I am sure you are excited to get started. The good thing is that you have a variety of intermittent fasting techniques that you can choose. In the following chapters, we will look at 7 intermittent fasting techniques and how to choose one that is best suited for your needs.

5. INTERMITTENT FASTING TECHNIQUES

The reason why fasting works for many dieters is because it has different techniques and can also be modified to suit any lifestyle. All approved methods of intermittent fasting stipulate how long you'd fast and the recommended diet to adapt during the feeding phase. As a beginner in fasting, you simply need to consider your current lifestyle and personal goals before you decide the type of intermittent fasting to adapt. Though there are many techniques to follow, lets discus seven of the most popular intermittent fasting techniques and how each of them works:

1. Alternate-Day Fasting

This diet suits disciplined eaters who have a specific goal weight. Created by James Johnson, the plan recommends that dieters eat a little amount of food or no food for 1 day and then eat normally the following day.

The diet works on the belief that alternating calorie intake can activate the SIRT1 gene, which boots fat metabolism and inhibits storage of fat. If on low calorie diet, let's say

Intermittent Fasting: 7 Effective Techniques with scientific approach

that of 2,000 calories daily, then you should eat 1/5th of your daily calories the first day. This translated to around 400 calories, which is a significant calorie cut especially for beginners.

To fight hunger during low-calorie days, you can opt for meal replacement shakes that are rich in essential nutrients. Try sipping the shakes in the entire day as opposed to splitting them into smaller meals. These shakes are however restricted to the first 2 days of the diet, to help you get adapted to low-calorie diet. For those who workout, you can reduce your weight-lifting exercises if you find it harder to hit the gym on the low calorie days, or save the sweat sessions for the normal calorie days.

According to reports, alternate day fasting can help you lose about 2 1/2 pounds of weight in a week especially if you cut calories intake by **20 to 35 percent. However, critics argue that as the diet is easy to follow, it can motivate dieters to binge eat on "normal eating"** days. If that's your worry, you can control binge eating on normal calorie days by scheduling meals beforehand, in order to meet the goal weight.

2. The Warrior Diet

Developed by Ori Hofmekler, the fasting plan is suited for people who like to follow strict rules, i.e. those dedicated or devoted. On this fasting plan, you are supposed to fast for 20 hours a day while training, and then eat one large meal at night. Actually, the creator of the diet was of the view that human beings are nocturnal eaters, specifically adapted to eat at night. While it may sound awkward, night eating is believed to help the body synthesize hormones and facilitate fat-burning during daytime. As opposed to many fasting plans, the warrior diet also recommends the type of foods to eat. Such dietary recommendations help you to feed the body with the nutrients it requires to be in sync with your circadian rhythms.

The initial fasting phase of the diet is concerned with 'under-eating' or not eating at all. However, for beginners, you can eat some raw veggies or fruits and a little protein during the 20 hours fast. This restricted eating is designed to maximize the flight response of your sympathetic nervous system, to boost energy, promote alertness and burn fat. After the 20-hours fast, you are allowed to eat; but you should begin with food groups such as veggies,

Intermittent Fasting: 7 Effective Techniques with scientific approach

the proteins and if need be eat fats much later. In case you finish the suggested food groups and you're not yet full, you are allowed to eat little amount of carbs. The 4 hours eating phase is designed to help the body to recover, and promote relaxation while absorbing the nutrients required for growth and repair.

The main advantage of warrior diet fasting plan is that you're allowed to eat a few snacks now and again so you can keep hunger at bay. And according to followers of the diet, you tend to achieve higher energy levels as well as increased fat loss. However, the strict diet plan can interfere with eating patterns especially if in places like social **gatherings. Those who don't like eating large meals late at night can find it harder to follow the guidelines on food to eat or eating in the order recommended.**

3. Eat Stop Eat Fasting Plan

Developed by Brad Pilon, the fasting plan basically targets healthy eaters who need an extra boost for weight loss. The plan revolves all about moderation i.e. you can eat all food types you want but in controlled amounts.

Intermittent Fasting: 7 Effective Techniques with scientific approach

Here you are required to fast for up to 24 hours 1-2 times a week, in what is referred to as "24 break from eating". During the fasting period, no eating food is allowed save for calorie-free beverages like water. Once the fasting period is concluded, you begin to eat normally without need to compensate for the time spent fasting. You can choose to break the fast with a big meal or just enjoy a healthy afternoon snack if this is what works for you. The timing is extremely flexible thus you can adjust it as per your preferences.

The Eat Stop Eat approach can help you reduce calorie intake without need to limit what you eat or count calories. Another benefit is that the plan is flexible in that you can start fasting for fewer hours than recommended 24 and then gradually increase the duration. For instance, you can begin the fast when busy; say on a day when you have no food or specific dinning obligations. Another benefit is that foods aren't restricted on the types of foods to eat or avoid, and that you don't have to count calories.

On the downside, you might find it difficult to manage 24 hours of fasting particularly when beginning the fasting. Within this period, you can experience mood changes and symptoms such as fatigue, headache, being anxious or sick especially for women. According to research, fasting can cause hormonal imbalance as starvation triggers hunger hormones and thus binge eating. It can also halt ovulation, stop menstrual cycle and reduce fertility by shrinking the ovaries. To some dieters, long period of dieting can make it more tempting to binge eat after fast and this can hamper weight loss.

However, you can improve body composition and lose weight with the plan, by including a number of workouts, especially resistance training. Another drawback is that though you can prevent binge eating (read over-eating), it requires self-control and usually takes time.

4. Lean-Gains Plan

As the name suggests, this fasting plan is designed to help gym goers who intend to loss body fat while building muscle. Created by Martain Berkhan, Lean-gains suggest that men should fast for 16 hours and women for about 14 hours daily.

In the fast period, you're not required to consume calories but there's an exception in sugar-free gum, diet soda, calorie-free sweeteners and black coffee preferably with a splash of milk. After breaking the fast, you can feed for the remaining 8-10 hours depending on your activity level.

The type of food to eat during the eating period largely depends on your workout, since you'll need higher carbs supply than fat when working out. However, protein content should be relatively higher say 1-1.5 grams of protein per body pound but this also depends on your activity level and gender.

As a starter, you may find it easier to fast from night to morning, and then continue with the fast 6 hours after bed. Although lean-gains plan can work for anyone or workout lifestyle, it's important to maintain a regular feeding window. While this may not seem important, it can help prevent your bodily hormones from getting off balance. While eating is not restricted, your calories must come from whole and unprocessed foods as these supply energy without causing sugar crashes. In some cases, you

can take a meal replacement bar or a little amount of protein shake that has no added sugars. As a beginner, you may find this plan favorable since you can eat at whichever time you choose and healthy food too within the feeding period. With a little patience, beginners can comfortably adapt to the lifestyle just like the ordinary 3 meals a day plan. However, lean-gains fasting plan has restrictions on what to eat particularly when working-out. While this helps to maximize muscle gains, some dieters find the plan strict especially when it comes to scheduling meals around workouts.

5. Fat Loss Forever

Just like the lean-gains, this fasting plan is designed to cater for gym goers who enjoy having a few cheat days. Designed by Dan Go and John Romaniello, the fasting plan allows you to enjoy a cheat day each week, although followed by a whopping 36 hours of fasting!

The diet work on the research finding that states that 36 hours of fasting boosts metabolism and accelerates weight loss. After the one-and-a half days of fasting, the remainder of 7-day cycle is divided between various fasting protocols.

For instance, you can choose Alternate Day Fasting or the Warriors Diet for that matter!

Intermittent Fasting: 7 Effective Techniques with scientific approach

This fat-loss fasting plan allows you to follow a 7-day program so that the body can achieve maximum fat loss. Particularly if on a busy program, the long fast facilitates you to focus on productivity and curb occasional cravings. If fasting for such long is hard for you, you can download or purchase training programs designed to help maximize fat loss. While having a cheat day could be a cool idea, it can motivate you to binge eat on unhealthy snacks that can hamper weight loss goals. Worse still, the plan suggests a 36-hour long fasting schedule that can be uncomfortable for most people.

6. The 5:2 Fast Diet

This is an easy to follow fasting plan that was coined by Michael Mosley, a British doctor and journalist. As its name suggests, it involves eating regularly for 5 days and then fasting for 2 days in a week.

On fasting day, women are required to eat 500 calories in a day while men are advised to consume 600 calories. The calories can be eaten any time of the day, whether as a single meal or spread in the entire day. You're also free to choose the days to fast as far as you involve at least one non-fasting day in between. For instance, you can decide to fast on Thursday and Monday while eating 2-3 small meals of up to 600 calories. You can eat foods such as soups as these enhance satiety and are low in calories compared to actual ingredients that make them. On normal eating days, focus on whole and healthy foods especially those with high protein and fiber to facilitate weight loss. Here you can eat natural yoghurt with berries, cauliflower rice, baked or boiled eggs, grilled meat, tea, black coffee or a generous portion of veggies. To come up with your fasting plan, you'll need to experiment whatever works for you.

7. The 2-Day Fast

As compared to other fasting plans where you fast for occasional 1 day, here you do a 2 days or 48-hour fast once every few months. This means that you'll need to go to bed hungry not for one day but for two full days!

While you could be scared of hunger, the body normally enters into nutritional ketosis where it burns stored fat for energy. To your surprise, once accustomed to the fast, you hardly become hungry as ketosis keeps you going. And if afraid of burning muscle, rest assured that increased fat metabolism and levels of HGH hormone will hinder muscle loss. For beginners, you may need to begin with a 24 hours fast before attempting the 2-day fast. Then ensure that you eat dinner the previous night say between 6-8 pm. After waking up the next morning, simply drink water to stay hydrated throughout the day. At 10 o'clock, drink a cup of green tea and later a cup of black coffee around noon, or instead take some mineral water. Ensure that you're busy the entire day and avoid encounter with foods that trigger cravings such as sweet snacks. Continue taking water until evening and then some decaf coffee or herbal tea for dinner. By now, you should be ready to fall asleep without feeling any hunger; and ready to progress with day two of fasting!   With practice, you'll find it easier to manage even longer than 48 hours of fasting without any negative side effects.   However, health experts warn that intermittent fasting is not for everyone. For this reason, you should consult a doctor before changing your diet patterns especially if you suffer from any health conditions. You also need to consider your current lifestyle and personal goals before you decide the type of intermittent fasting to adapt.

Intermittent Fasting: 7 Effective Techniques with scientific approach

To guide you on possible fasting plan to consider, these following tips can help a lot:

How to Choose Best Fasting Technique

If healthy, managing a fast is an easy thing as far as you can retrain your body to burn fat for fuel and lose weight. Since it harder to burn fat in cases where the body accesses other sources of fuel, you should choose a technique that focuses on fewer meals that are timed to occur closely together.

You also need to eat only the real foods when it comes to eating phase, say organic produce and pastured eggs, meat and dairy.

Any fasting technique can apply here as except Fat Loss Forever plan as it suggests that you include a few cheat days. Simply cut out any sugary or processed foods such as sweets, chocolate, crisps and fizzy drinks.

But when it comes to food choices, it's advisable to consume food groups based on the type of fasting you adopt. Start by slowly withdrawing from specific foods or simply replace them with healthier or low-calorie options. For instance, you can swap the shortening or butter with coconut oil and schedule those Pop-tarts for post-workout. Also stock healthy oatcakes, unsalted rice cakes, fruit juice, unsweetened popcorn and healthy fruits. After 2-3 weeks, you can then choose to eat at specific times, say from 10 a.m-8 p.m. Once accustomed with the eating plan, you can fully embark on 16-18 hours fasting plan or alternate day fasting.

The intermittent fasting technique that you choose should depend on your activity level, work program and the availability of food. For instance, body builders should choose Lean-Gains or Fast Loss Forever plans while non-gym goers can choose Eat Stop Diet or the 5:2 fasting plan. If busy throughout the day or unable to access food, you can try out the Warrior diet that promotes 4-hours night eating window. If ready to try something more challenging, then a 48-72 hour fasting can help you gain more in terms of weight loss. If seeking to lose weight, choose a fasting technique that can accommodate exercise. Alternatively, adopt a fitness program that is based on cardio, yoga or interval training. Being in a training program facilitates alternate periods of intense activity with bursts of slower recovery. To begin with, try 20-30 minutes of bike riding, walking or swimming to rev your metabolism and thus burn more calories. With interval training, you can develop leaner muscles to further rev the metabolism; to assist you break that weight loss plateau.

Regardless of the fasting technique that you choose, it's recommendable to not eat food but rather drink plenty of water, tea and coffee to remain hydrated. Water can serve as a good substitute for occasional snacks as it contains no calories or added sugars. To help sweeten and make water tasty, consider adding a little amount of stevia or lemon juice. Water also helps you remain hydrated and supercharges various metabolic activities among them digestion and removal of toxins from your body. In case you find it easier to fast for 2-3 weeks, consider fasting more often preferably fasting longer on weekends.

So how can you easily succeed with intermittent fasting? These 4 guidelines can be much helpful:

6. TIPS TO SUCCEED WITH FASTING & CONCLUSION

Intermittent Fasting: 7 Effective Techniques with scientific approach

1. Don't start too ambitious

It's a hard thing to transit from binge eating or following a regular diet of junk food into a few meals in a day or no meal at all for 1-2 days. Even for dieters who now eat one meal in a day, remember they never started like that. You need to first skip your breakfast or dinner, do without lunch for at least 16 hours or 20 hours of fast.

Do not be too harsh on yourself, and don't' be overly ambitious. While it may appear easy to first, a few of dieters take days or weeks to manage a 24-48 hours of total fasting.

Also know that setting short-term achievable goals can play a big role in fighting stress that may interrupt your progress. A short term goal may include something like a lean and healthy breakfast every day within one week.

2. Don't be afraid of hunger

Understand that hunger is totally a normal part of life and that a few hours of fast can't eat away your muscles. Even with 16-48 hours of fast, you can still manage ordinary workout routines and build bigger muscles.

Furthermore, you don't have to worry on which time you eat food as far as it's within the feeding window. Some dieters eat a single meal in a day at around 3-4 pm, a meal that serves as dinner and then survive on water and tea.

In case you feel hungry before or after dinner, try eating few raw veggies or some bit of ice cream.

3. Cope with cravings

In those instances when food cravings strike, just appreciate them without allowing yourself to get distracted or rather fulfill them. Try getting yourself busy through trying out a more involving task, visit your friend or go for a walk.

Cravings do go away within 15-60 minutes of getting into more productive ventures. If not successful, take a few satiating drinks such as soups, water or tea and then consider eating more veggies during the feeding window. Veggies are delicious and tasty when served with brown rice or other whole food. Choose high fiber veggies topped with whole grains to fight hunger.

Such dietary combination also helps to slow down the absorption of glucose into your blood.

4. Get enough nutrients

You can also take multivitamins or 5-8 grams of amino acids such as branched chain amino acids (BCAAs). These support weight loss by strengthening your body cells and muscles, bones and supplying required energy. For instance, vitamin B helps your body cells make protein, release energy and to manufacture serotonin, a brain chemical. Get vitamin B from fat-free dairy products, soy products, salmon, sardines, lean meat, eggs and fat-free peanut butter.

With these tips and strong will at heart, you can surely overcome any barrier as far as fasting is concerned. But in case you develop negative hormonal imbalance symptoms such as fatigue, headaches, bloating, depression or irregular periods, stop fasting. It's wise to do so as such symptoms may accelerate it to an eating disorder or other serious condition.

Conclusion

Tip: To effectively burn fat and build muscle, carb cycling can really be helpful so you can find a blend of intermittent fasting and carb cycling. When carb intake is low, the body is forced to use body fat as source of energy. However, the body still require specific amount of carbs to facilitate nervous and brain functions. Thus for gym goers, try to up the carb intake to at least 50 grams to replenish your glycogen stores. Ensure that you consume enough amounts of proteins and fats while not limiting intake of carbohydrates below 50 grams. With the correct approach, you should reap benefits of intermittent fasting within no time!

....

Hey! Do you mind giving your feedback on Amazon by rating and reviewing my book.

I would really appreciate that.

....

My Other Books available across the platforms in e-book, paperback and audible versions:

1. Love Yourself: 21 day plan for learning "Self-Love" to cultivate self-worth ,self-belief, self-confidence & happiness

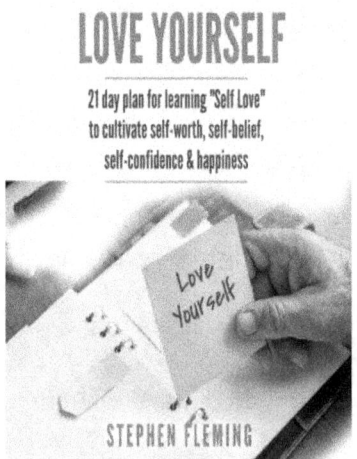

2. Intermittent Fasting: 7 effective techniques of Intermittent Fasting

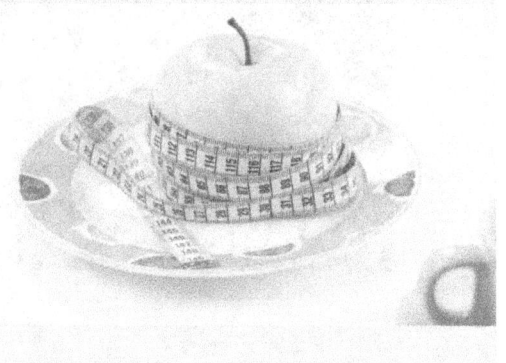

3. Blockchain Technology : Introduction to Blockchain Technology and its impact on Business Ecosystem

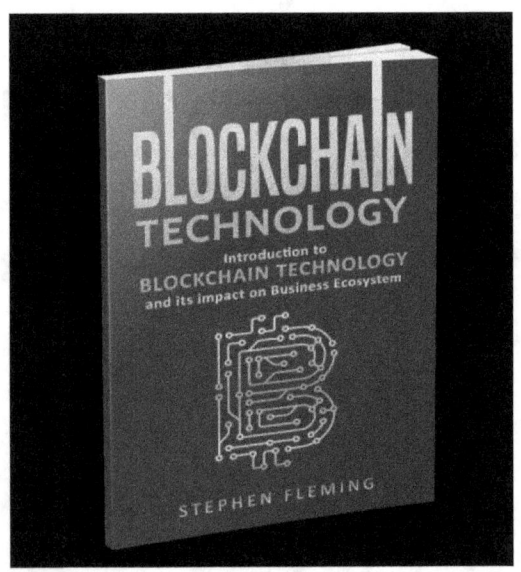

4. DevOps Handbook: Introduction to DevOps and its impact on Business Ecosystem

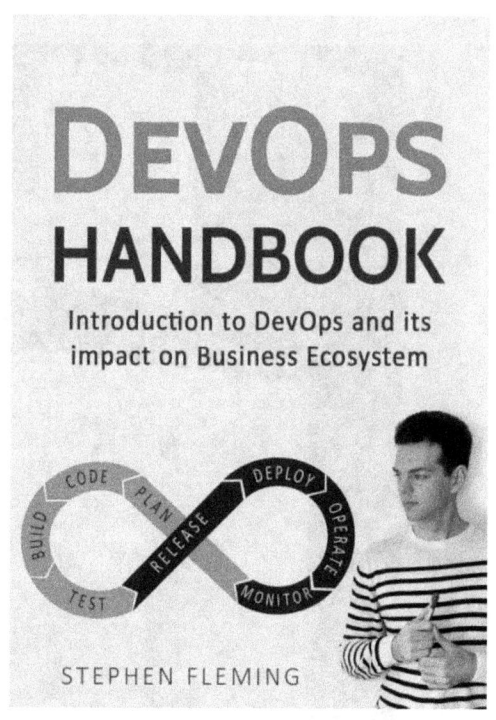

5. Blockchain Technology & DevOps: Introduction and impact on Business Ecosystem

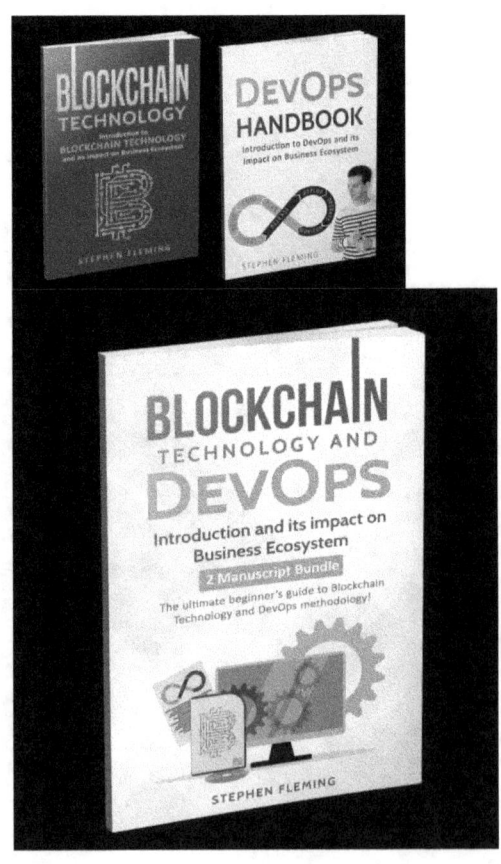

** If you prefer audible versions of these books, I have few free coupons, drop me a mail at: valueadd2life@gmail.com. If available, I would mail you the same.

www.ingramcontent.com/pod-product-compliance
Lightning Source LLC
LaVergne TN
LVHW011900060526
838200LV00054B/4452